THE CRPS COOKBOOK

HEALTHY NUTRITION FOR MANAGING PAINS OF STINGING AND TEARING SENSATION

KAREN EDMONDS

TABLE OF CONTENT

STAY
HEALTHY

INTRODUCTION

Welcome to "The CRPS Cookbook," your go-to resource for creating tasty and health-conscious meals for people living with Complex Regional Pain Syndrome (CRPS). In this cookbook, we will explore how a well-balanced and thoughtfully designed food might help alleviate the problems offered by CRPS.

Living with CRPS requires special nutritional considerations, and this cookbook is intended to be your food preparation partner, providing easy and accessible dishes that prioritise nutrition without sacrificing flavour. Our objective is to provide you with information regarding CRPS and nutrition basics, allowing you to make more educated dietary choices.

Within these pages, you will find a range of breakfast pleasures, lunchtime favourites, and supper alternatives that not only satisfy your cravings but also adhere to CRPS-friendly dietary standards. From creating a CRPS-friendly pantry to adopting mindful eating habits, this cookbook seeks to make your path to heath both fun and accessible.

Whether you are an experienced home cook or just starting out, "The CRPS Cookbook" will inspire and encourage you in producing meals that promote your general well-being. Let us go on this delightful and fulfilling journey together.

CHAPTER 1: OVERVIEW OF CRPS

Complex Regional Pain Syndrome (CRPS) is a chronic pain disease marked by significant, ongoing pain that is out of proportion to the initial injury or trauma. It usually affects one arm or leg, but it can occur anywhere on the body. The specific aetiology of CRPS is unknown, however it typically occurs after an accident, surgery, or trauma.

CRPS causes a wide range of sensory and autonomic symptoms. Intense, searing pain is a defining feature, which might be accompanied by increased sensitivity to touch or temperature changes. Common autonomic symptoms include swelling, changes in skin colour or temperature, and excessive sweating or dryness in the afflicted region.

People with CRPS may suffer changes in skin texture, such as thinning or shine, as well as joint stiffness. Motor symptoms such as muscular spasms, tremors, or weakness may also occur. The pain and symptoms of CRPS can cause substantial impairment and interfere with regular activities.

Seeking medical attention is critical for an accurate diagnosis and developing a complete treatment plan that may include pain medication, physical therapy, and psychological support to enhance the overall quality of life for those with CRPS.

Importance of a Healthy and Balanced Diet for CRPS Management

Maintaining a healthy and balanced diet is critical in controlling Complex Regional Pain Syndrome (CRPS). A well-nourished body adds to general health and can improve numerous elements of CRPS therapy.

Pain Reduction: Certain foods include anti-inflammatory characteristics that may help decrease CRPS discomfort. A diet high in fruits, vegetables, healthy grains, and fatty fish might help to lower inflammation, thereby alleviating discomfort.

Tissue Repair and Maintenance: CRPS frequently causes changes in skin, muscles, and bones. Adequate nutritional consumption, including vitamins and minerals, promotes tissue repair and maintenance, hence improving overall physical well-being.

Weight Management: Keeping a healthy weight is critical for those with CRPS. Excess weight might worsen discomfort and tension in afflicted limbs. A balanced diet, along with regular physical activity as prescribed by healthcare specialists, can help with weight control.

Energy and stamina: CRPS can be physically demanding, and people may feel fatigued. A well-balanced diet gives the energy required to carry out everyday tasks, lowering the influence of exhaustion on quality of life.

Mood and Mental Health: Nutrient-rich diets can help improve mental health. A well-balanced diet can assist to stabilise blood sugar levels, which in turn helps to regulate mood and lessen anxiety or depression symptoms that are frequently connected with chronic pain disorders.

Optimal Bone Health: CRPS can occasionally impair bone density. Adequate calcium and vitamin D consumption, either through food or supplements as prescribed by healthcare specialists, can assist to maintain good bone health.

Gut Health: Some people with CRPS may develop gastrointestinal problems. A diet high in fibre, probiotics, and easily digested foods can support gut health and perhaps relieve digestive disorders.

Incorporating these dietary concepts into a complete CRPS management plan, together with medical treatments and therapies, improves the overall well-being of those dealing with this difficult illness. Individuals must collaborate with healthcare specialists, particularly dietitians, to customise dietary advice based on their unique requirements and symptoms.

EAT HEALTHY AND BE HAPPY

CHAPTER 2: NUTRITIONAL GUIDELINES FOR CRPS

Nutritional advice for people with Complex Regional Pain Syndrome (CRPS) are centred on boosting general health, regulating inflammation, and treating probable nutritional shortages. Individual needs may differ, however the following basic recommendations can be considered:

Anti-inflammatory Foods:

Encourage a diet high in fruits and vegetables, which contain antioxidants that help fight inflammation.

Fatty fish such as salmon, mackerel, and sardines contain omega-3 fatty acids, which are recognised for their anti-inflammatory qualities.

Balanced Macronutrients:

Maintain a mix of carbs, proteins, and healthy fats to boost energy and nutrition.

Choose whole grains, lean meats, and healthy fats like avocados, almonds, and olive oil.

Vitamins and Minerals:

Consume a variety of nutrient-dense meals to get enough vitamins and minerals.

Pay attention to calcium and vitamin D for bone health, especially if CRPS impairs movement.

Hydration:

Stay hydrated by drinking water and other hydrating beverages. Proper hydration improves joint health and general body function.

Limit processed foods:

Reduce your consumption of processed foods, which may include chemicals and preservatives that might worsen inflammation.

Mindful eating:

Pay attention to hunger and fullness indicators to cultivate mindful eating skills. This technique can help you develop a balanced connection with food and avoid overeating.

Food Sensitivity Awareness:

Be aware of any dietary sensitivities or triggers that may worsen CRPS symptoms. Keeping a food journal might aid in determining likely culprits.

Small, frequent meals:

Consider eating smaller, more frequent meals to keep a consistent energy level and avoid putting undue strain on the digestive system.

Collaboration with Health Professionals:

Collaborate with healthcare specialists, including dietitians, to create a personalised nutrition plan based on your specific requirements and symptoms.

Supplementation, if necessary:

Consider supplements to treat any diagnosed nutritional deficiencies, as advised by your doctor. This might include vitamins, minerals, or omega-3 supplements.

Individuals with CRPS should work with a healthcare provider to adjust these instructions to their unique health state and need. A personalised and comprehensive strategy that combines diet, medical care, and lifestyle changes can help people with CRPS improve their overall well-being.

Building a CRPS-Friendly Pantry

Building a CRPS-friendly pantry entails choosing items that promote general health, reduce inflammation, and address the specific dietary needs associated with Complex Regional Pain Syndrome. Here is how to fill your pantry with CRPS-friendly options:

Whole grains:

Choose whole grains such as brown rice, quinoa, muesli and whole wheat pasta. These give complex carbs and fibre for long-lasting energy.

Lean proteins:

Choose lean proteins such skinless chicken, fish, tofu, lentils, and beans. Protein is essential for muscle function and repair.

Healthy fats:

Include sources of healthy fats such as avocados, nuts, seeds, and olive oil. These lipids are anti-inflammatory and promote general well-being.

Canned or frozen vegetables:

Keep canned or frozen veggies on hand for quick and simple meal additions. They keep their nutritious value and provide convenience.

Canned legumes:

Stock up on canned legumes such as chickpeas, black beans, and lentils. They are adaptable, protein-rich, and may be used into a variety of meals.

Low sodium broths and soups:

Use low-sodium broths and soups as the foundation for nutritional meals. They enhance flavour and may be customised with extra ingredients.

Herbs and spices:

Use herbs and spices to enhance the flavour of your food. Turmeric, ginger, garlic, and cinnamon, for example, have anti-inflammatory compounds.

Healthy sweeteners:

Rather with processed sugars, use natural sweeteners such as honey, maple syrup, or agave nectar. These alternatives can be used in moderation to achieve sweetness.

Gluten-Free Options (where needed):

If you are sensitive to gluten, consider gluten-free options. Gluten-free pasta, rice flour, and oats are all available.

Nutrient-Rich Snacks:

Keep nutritious snacks on available, such as mixed nuts, dried fruits, and whole-grain crackers. These might be useful and satisfying in between meals.

Alternative Flours:

Consider using alternative flours such as almond flour, coconut flour, or chickpea flour for baking or cooking. These may be good for persons with dietary restrictions.

Hydrating beverages:

To promote general hydration, stock your pantry with hydrating beverages such as herbal teas, flavoured water, and electrolyte-rich drinks.

Assess and update your pantry on a regular basis, taking into account your food choices, nutritional requirements, and any modifications to your CRPS management plan. Consult with healthcare specialists or a certified dietitian to fine-tune your pantry options depending on your specific health needs.

Reading Food Labels for CRPS-Friendly Choices:

Check for additives and preservatives:

Avoid items that have too many additives, preservatives, or artificial colours, since they may lead to inflammation.

Be mindful of sodium content:

To limit sodium consumption, use canned foods with little or no added salt. This can alter inflammation and fluid retention.

Select Whole Foods:

To maximise nutritional advantages, aim for minimally processed, whole foods rather than highly processed choices.

Look for whole grains:

Check product labels for whole grains as the principal ingredient, which guarantees a greater fibre content.

Consider sugar content:

To promote general health, be mindful of added sugars in goods and choose for reduced sugar choices.

Review Allergen Information:

If you have food sensitivities or allergies, read allergy information thoroughly to prevent potential triggers.

By proactively stocking up on these critical components and paying attention to product labels, you may establish a pantry that meets your nutritional needs while also assisting in the treatment of CRPS symptoms. Consult a healthcare practitioner or a qualified dietician for personalised advice based on your individual health needs.

Substituting Ingredients for a Healthier Twist:

Substituting healthier components into your meals is an excellent approach to make them more CRPS-friendly while also contributing to your general well-being. Here are some recommendations for food swaps that improve nutritional value while maintaining flavour:

Flour:

Replace refined white flour with whole wheat flour, almond flour, coconut flour, or oat flour to increase fibre and nutrition.

Sweeteners:

Replace processed sugars with natural sweeteners like honey, maple syrup, or agave nectar for a hint of sweetness and potential health benefits.

Cooking Oils:

Choose better cooking oils such as olive oil, avocado oil, or coconut oil over vegetable oils for heart-healthy monounsaturated fats.

Dairy:

Choose dairy substitutes such as almond milk, coconut milk, or soy milk to lower your saturated fat consumption, especially if you are lactose intolerant.

Salt:

Instead of using too much salt, season your foods with herbs, spices, and citrus juice. This helps to regulate salt intake, potentially lowering inflammation and fluid retention.

Protein:

To maintain muscle without adding saturated fats, choose lean protein sources such as skinless poultry, fish, tofu, or lentils over processed or fatty meats.

Grains:

Replace refined grains with whole grains such as brown rice, quinoa, or barley for more fibre and minerals.

Snacks:

For a healthier and more enjoyable snack, choose nutrient-dense options such as fresh fruit, mixed nuts, or air-popped popcorn over processed alternatives.

Dressing and sauces:

Make your homemade dressings with olive oil, balsamic vinegar, and herbs instead of buying store-bought ones with added sweets and bad fats.

Desserts:

Use mashed bananas, applesauce, or yoghurt as natural sweeteners and moisture enhancers in baking to reduce the need for additional sugars and fats.

Pasta:

Consider whole wheat or alternate grain pasta for more fibre and nutrients than standard white pasta.

Sodium-free broths:

Choose low-sodium or sodium-free broths for soups and stews to reduce sodium consumption without sacrificing flavour.

BE

HAPPY

CHAPTER 3: BREAKFAST DELIGHTS

Açaí Smoothie Bowl

Açaí Smoothie Bowl

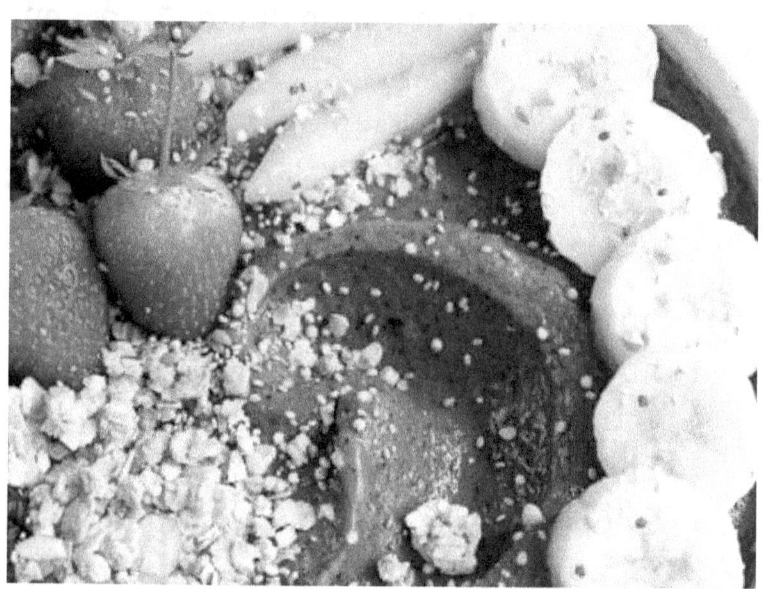

Ingredients:

Açaí Smoothie Base:

- 1 pack (100 grams) frozen unsweetened açaí berries

- 1/2 frozen banana
- 1/2 cup of frozen mixed berries (blueberries, strawberries, raspberries)
- 1/2 cup of unsweetened almond milk (or any milk of choice)
- 1 tablespoon of chia seeds
- 1 tablespoon of almond butter or peanut butter
- 1 tablespoon of honey or maple syrup (optional for sweetness)

Toppings:

- Sliced banana
- Fresh berries(blueberries, strawberries)
- Granola or muesli
- Shredded coconut
- Chopped nuts (almonds, walnuts, or your preference)

Preparation:

Blend the Açaí Smoothie Base:

- Combine frozen açaí berries, frozen banana, mixed berries, almond milk, chia seeds, almond butter, and honey or

maple syrup (optional) in a blender.
Blend until you get a thick, silky consistency. If required, add additional almond milk to get the desired consistency.

Assemble the Bowl:

- Pour the açaí smoothie in a bowl.
  Add toppings:
  Place sliced banana, fresh berries, granola, shredded coconut, and chopped almonds on top of the smoothie base.

Drizzle with honey or peanut butter:

- Drizzle with additional honey or add a dollop of nut butter for more sweetness and richness.

Enjoy:

- Enjoy with a spoon the delightful combination of açaí goodness and vivid toppings.

Nutritional Value (approx. per serving):

Calories: 400-450 kcal

Protein: 10-15g

Fat: 20-25g

Carbohydrates: 50-60g

Dietary Fibre: 10-15g

Sugar: 25-30g

Notes

Your

Observation

Oatmeal Cookie Overnight Oats

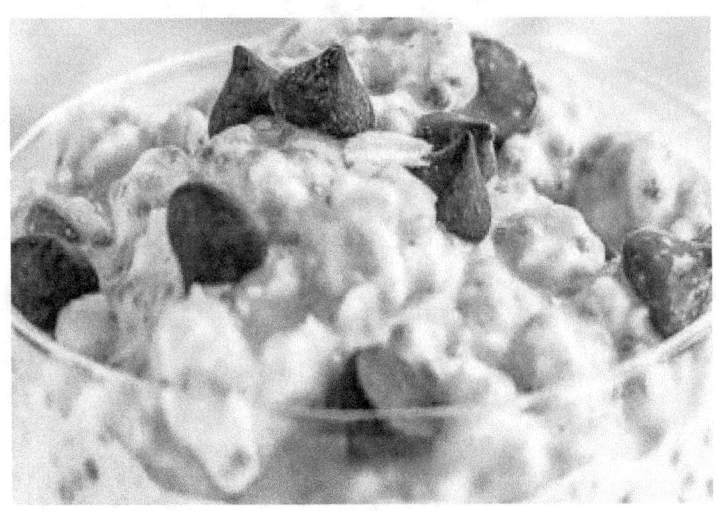

Ingredients:

Base:

- 1/2 cup of rolled oats
- 1/2 cup of milk of your choice (dairy or plant-based)
- 1/2 cup of Greek yogurt (or dairy-free alternative for a vegan option)

- 1 tablespoon of chia seeds
- 1/2 teaspoon of vanilla extract

Flavour Enhancers:

- 1 tablespoon of almond butter or peanut butter
- 1 tablespoon of honey or maple syrup (adjust to taste)
- 1/4 teaspoon of cinnamon
- Pinch of salt

Additional Mix-Ins (for cookie-like texture):

- 1 tablespoon of raisins
- 1 tablespoon of chopped nuts (walnuts, almonds, or pecans)

Toppings (optional):

- Sliced bananas
- Additional drizzle of honey or nut butter

Preparation:

Combine Base Ingredients:

- In a container, combine rolled oats, milk, Greek yoghurt, chia seeds, vanilla essence, almond butter, honey or maple syrup, cinnamon, and a pinch of salt.
- Stir carefully to ensure all components are well blended. Stir until smooth and the oats are well covered.

Add Mix-Ins:

- Gently mix in raisins and chopped nuts to achieve the oatmeal cookie texture.

Refrigerate:

- Refrigerate overnight or at least 4 hours to let the oats absorb the liquid and flavours.

Serve:

- Before serving, mix the oats well. If the mixture is too thick, add a splash of milk to get the correct consistency.
- Optional toppings for this oatmeal cookie-inspired breakfast include sliced bananas, honey, or nut butter.

Nutritional Value (approx. per serving):

Calories: 400-450 kcal

Protein: 15-20g

Fat: 15-20g

Carbohydrates: 50-60g

Dietary Fibre: 8-10g

Sugar: 20-25g

Notes

Your

Observation

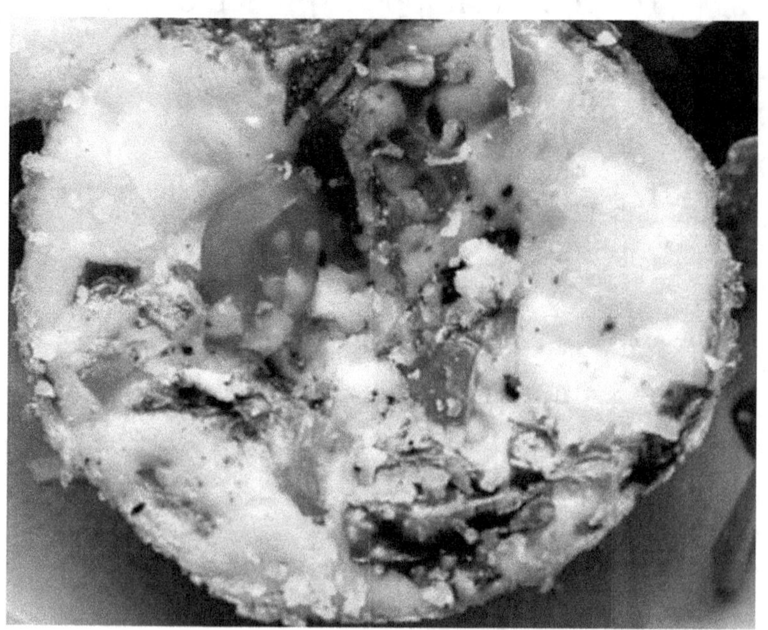

Ingredients:

Base:

- 6 big eggs
- 1/2 cup of milk (dairy or plant-based)
- Salt and pepper, to taste

Vegetables:

- 1/2 cup of diced bell peppers
- 1/2 cup of diced tomatoes
- 1/2 cup of chopped spinach or kale
- 1/4 cup of diced red onions

Protein:

- 1/2 cup of cooked and crumbled turkey sausage or diced ham (optional)

Cheese:

- 1/2 cup of shredded cheddar, feta, or your preferred cheese

Herbs and Spices:

- 1 teaspoon of dried oregano or Italian seasoning
- 1/2 teaspoon of garlic powder

Preparation:

Preheat the Oven:

- Preheat the oven to 350°F (175° C). Grease a muffin tray or use silicone or parchment paper liners.

- Whisk In a bowl, mix together eggs, milk, salt, and pepper until thoroughly blended.

Prepare vegetables:

- Dice the bell peppers, tomatoes, and red onions. Chop spinach or kale.

Sauté Vegetables:

- Sauté diced vegetables in a pan over medium heat until slightly softened. Set aside for cooling.

Combine   ingredients:

- Incorporate sautéed vegetables, crumbled sausage or ham, grated cheese, dry oregano and garlic powder into the egg mixture. Stir until well blended.

Fill Muffin Cups:

- To fill muffin cups, evenly distribute the mixture and leave enough room at the top for the frittatas to expand while baking.

Bake:

- Bake in a preheated oven for 20-25 minutes, or until the tops are gently brown.

Serve:

- To serve, let frittata muffins cool in the muffin tray for a few minutes before transferring to a wire rack. Serve warm or room temperature.

Nutritional Value (approx. per serving):

Calories: 120-150 kcal per muffin

Protein: 10-12g

Fat: 7-9g

Carbohydrates: 3-5g

Fibre: 1-2g

Sugar: 1-2g

Notes

Your Observation

EMBRACE POSITIVITY

CHAPTER 4: LUNCH FAVOURITES

Gluten-Free Mujaddara

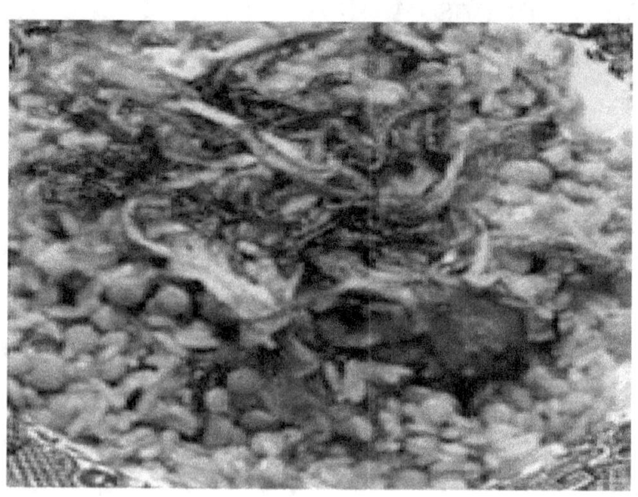

Ingredients:

Base:

- 1 cup of gluten-free green or brown lentils, washed and drained

- 1 cup of gluten-free rice (such as basmati), washed and drained
- 3 cups of water
- 1 big onion, thinly sliced

Seasonings:

- 3 tablespoons of olive oil
- 1 teaspoon of ground cumin
- 1 teaspoon of ground coriander
- 1/2 teaspoon of crushed cinnamon
- Salt and pepper, to taste

Optional Toppings:

- Yogurt or dairy-free yogurt
- Fresh parsley, chopped
- Pomegranate seeds

Preparation:

Prepare Lentils and Rice:

- Mix the lentils, rice, and water in a large saucepan. Bring to a boil, then decrease heat to low, cover, and cook until lentils and rice are soft and water has been absorbed (approximately 20-25 minutes).

Caramelise onions:

- To caramelise onions, heat 2 tablespoons olive oil in a pan over medium heat while the lentils and rice simmer. Add the thinly sliced onions and heat, stirring periodically, until golden brown and caramelised. Set aside.

Season mujaddara:

- To season the Mujaddara, add the remaining one tablespoon olive oil to the skillet. Stir in the ground cumin, coriander, cinnamon, salt, and pepper. Cook for 1-2 minutes, until the spices are fragrant.

Combine Ingredients:

- Cook lentils and rice first, then add the spicy onion combination. Gently combine everything, allowing the flavours to mingle. Adjust the salt and pepper to taste.

Serve:

- Move the gluten-free mujaddara to a serving plate. Top with caramelised onions and optional ingredients like as yoghurt, fresh parsley, and pomegranate seeds.

Enjoy:

- This gluten-free version of mujaddara is a tasty and fulfilling main dish or side dish. Serve warm.

Nutritional Value (approx. per serving):

Calories: 300-350 kcal per serving

Protein: 10-15g

Fat: 8-10g

Carbohydrates: 50-60g

Dietary Fibre: 8-10g

Sugar: 2-3g

Notes

Your

Observation

Crispy Potatoes with Kefir and Vegetables

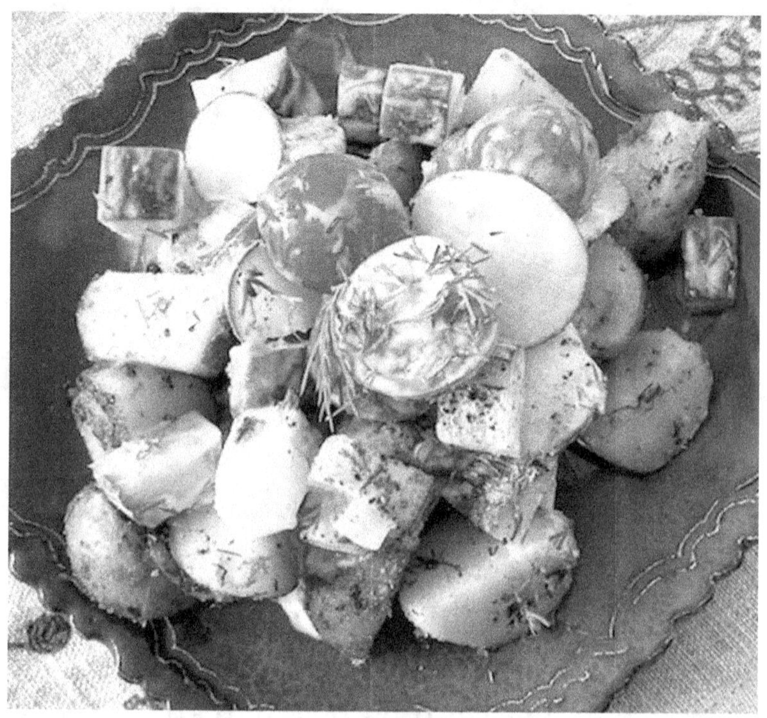

Ingredients:

Potatoes:

- 4 big potatoes, peeled and diced into eatable pieces
- 2 tablespoons of olive oil
- Salt and pepper, to taste
- 1 teaspoon of paprika (optional, for extra flavor)

Kefir Dressing:

- 1 cup of kefir (dairy or non-dairy)
- 2 tablespoons of olive oil
- 1 clove of minced garlic
- 1 tablespoon of lemon juice
- Salt and pepper, to taste

Vegetables:

- 1 bell pepper, thinly sliced
- 1 zucchini, thinly sliced
- 1 red onion, thinly sliced
- 1 cup cherry tomatoes, halved
- Fresh herbs for garnish (parsley, chives, or mint)

Preparation:

Crispy Potatoes:

- Preheat the oven to 425° Fahrenheit (220° Celsius).
- Combine chopped potatoes, olive oil, salt, pepper, and paprika (if using) in a mixing dish.
- Place the potatoes on a baking pan in a single layer. Bake for 30-35 minutes, or until golden and crispy. Flip halfway through.

Prepare the Kefir Dressing:

- In a small mixing bowl, combine kefir, olive oil, chopped garlic, lemon juice, salt, and pepper. Adjust the seasoning to your liking.

Sauté vegetables:

- While the potatoes are baking, heat a little olive oil in a pan over medium heat. Add the sliced red pepper, zucchini and red onion. Sauté the vegetables for 5-7 minutes, until they are soft yet still crisp. Remove from heat.

Assemble:

- When the potatoes are crispy and golden, place them on a serving platter. Arrange the sautéed vegetables on top.
- Drizzle Kefir Dressing over Crispy Potatoes and Vegetables.
- Garnish with half cherry tomatoes and fresh herbs of choice.

Serve:

- Serve the crispy potatoes with kefir and vegetables right away to maximise their crispiness and flavour.

Nutritional Value (approx. per serving):

Calories: 300-350 kcal

Protein: 8-10g

Fat: 15-20g

Carbohydrates: 35-40g

Dietary Fibre: 5-7g

Sugar: 5-7g

Notes

Your

Observation

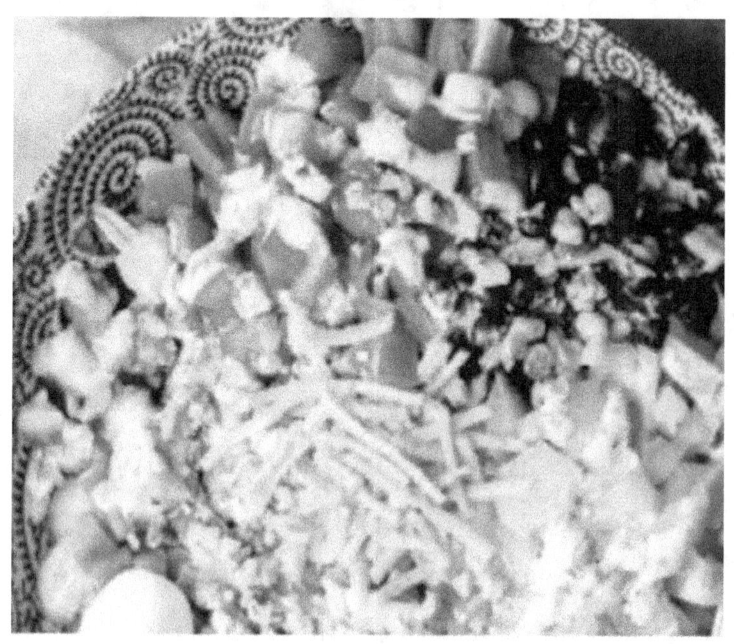

Ingredients:

Salad:

- 1 cup of cooked quinoa

- 1 can (15 oz) chickpeas, washed and drained
- 1 cucumber, chopped
- 1 cup of cherry tomatoes, halved
- 1 red bell pepper, diced
- 1/2 red onion, thinly chopped
- 1/4 cup of Kalamata olives, sliced
- 1/4 cup of feta cheese, crumbled (optional)
- Fresh parsley, chopped, for garnish

Dressing:

- 3 tablespoons of extra-virgin olive oil
- 2 tablespoons of balsamic vinegar
- 1 teaspoon of Dijon mustard
- 1 clove of minced garlic
- Salt and pepper, to taste

Preparations:

Prepare Quinoa and Chickpeas:

- Cook the quinoa according to the package directions and let it cool.

- Mix the cooked quinoa and chickpeas in a big bowl.

Chop vegetables:

- Mix in the chopped cucumber, cherry tomatoes, red bell pepper, red onion, Kalamata olives, and feta cheese (if using) to the quinoa and chickpea combination.

Make the dressing:

- In a small bowl, combine the olive oil, balsamic vinegar, Dijon mustard, minced garlic, salt, and pepper.

Prepare the Salad:

- Pour the dressing over the salad and gently toss to cover everything evenly.

Garnish and serve:

- Garnish the salad with fresh parsley and serve immediately. Alternatively, chill for a few hours to allow the flavours to combine before serving.

Nutritional Value (approx. per serving):

Calories: 350-400 kcal per serving

Protein: 12-15g

Fat: 15-20g

Carbohydrates: 45-50g

Dietary Fibre: 8-10g

Sugar: 7-9g

Notes

Your

Observation

Mediterranean Chicken Wrap

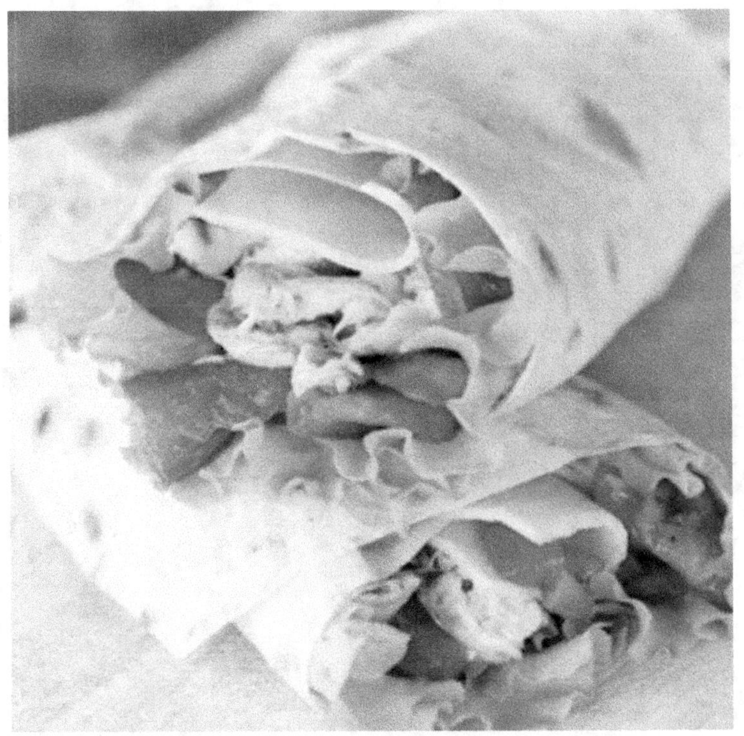

Ingredients:

For the Chicken:

- 2 boneless, skinless chicken breasts
- 1 tablespoon of olive oil

- 1 teaspoon of dried oregano
- 1 teaspoon of garlic powder
- Salt and pepper, to taste

For the Wrap:

- 4 big whole wheat or spinach tortillas
- 1 cup of hummus
- 1 cup of young spinach leaves
- 1/2 cup of sliced cucumber
- 1/2 cup of sliced cherry tomatoes
- 1/4 cup of sliced red onion
- 1/4 cup of crumbled feta cheese
- Kalamata olives, pitted and sliced (optional)
- Tzatziki sauce, for serving (optional)

Preparations:

Prepare the Chicken:

- Season the chicken breasts with olive oil, dried oregano, garlic powder, salt, and pepper.

- Preheat a grill pan or skillet to medium-high heat. Cook the chicken breasts for 6-7 minutes on each side, or until thoroughly done. Let them rest for a few minutes before slicing thinly.

Assemble the Wrap:

- Arrange each tortilla on a clean surface.
  Spread 1/4 cup hummus over each tortilla, leaving a border around the borders.

Add the fillings:

- Spread sliced chicken, baby spinach leaves, sliced cucumber, cherry tomatoes, red onion, crumbled feta cheese, and sliced Kalamata olives (if using) equally on each tortilla.

Roll up the wrap:

- Fold in the tortilla's sides and wrap it up firmly from the bottom to surround the ingredients.

Serve:

- Cut the wraps in half diagonally and serve right once, or wrap firmly in foil or parchment paper for a portable lunch.
  Optional: Serve with tzatziki sauce. Serve the wraps with a side of tzatziki sauce to dip into or drizzle over the contents before wrapping.

Nutritional Value (approx. per serving):

Calories: 400-450 kcal per wrap

Protein: 25-30g

Fat: 15-20g

Carbohydrates: 40-45g

Dietary Fibre: 6-8g

Sugar: 5-7g

Notes

Your
Observation

CHAPTER 5: DINNER DELIGHT

Baked Salmon with Dill Sauce

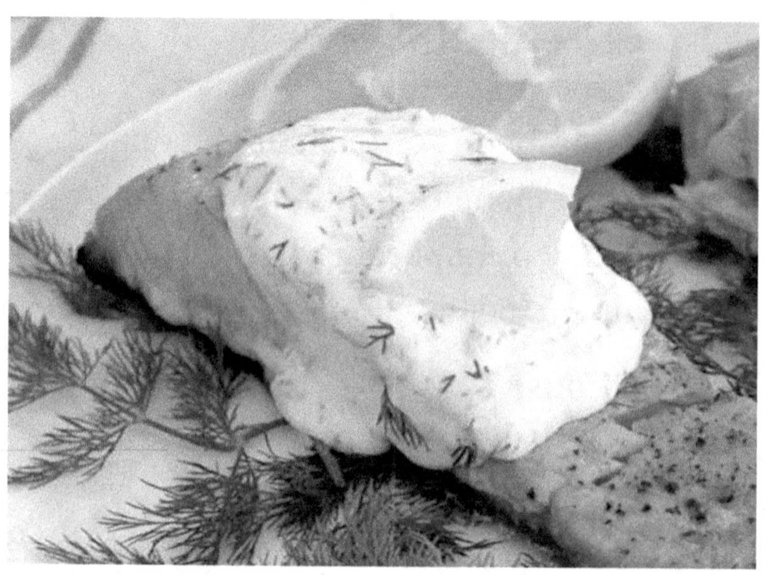

Ingredients:

For the Salmon:

- 4 salmon fillets (about 6 ounces each)
- 2 tablespoons of olive oil

- Salt and pepper, to taste
- 1 lemon, sliced (for garnish)
- Fresh dill sprigs (for garnish)

For the Dill Sauce:

- 1/2 cup of plain Greek yogurt
- 2 tablespoons of mayonnaise
- 1 tablespoon of Dijon mustard
- 2 tablespoons of fresh dill, chopped
- 1 tablespoon of lemon juice
- 1 clove of minced garlic
- Salt and pepper, to taste

Preparations:

Preheat the Oven:

- Preheat the oven to 400 °F (200 °C). To make cleaning easier, line a baking sheet with parchment paper or foil.

Prepare the salmon:

- Pat the salmon fillets dry with paper towels. Brush olive oil on both sides of each fillet and season with salt and pepper.

Bake the salmon:

- Place the salmon fillets on the prepared baking sheet, evenly spaced. If using skin-on salmon, place it skin side down.
- Bake in the preheated oven for 12-15 minutes, or until the salmon is fully cooked and easily flaked with a fork. Cooking time varies according to the thickness of the fillets.

Make the dill sauce:

- While the salmon bakes, make the dill sauce. In a small mixing bowl, combine the Greek yoghurt, mayonnaise, Dijon mustard, chopped dill, lemon juice, minced garlic, salt, and pepper. Whisk until smooth. Season to taste.

Serve:

- After the salmon has cooked, transfer it to serving plates. Drizzle each fillet with a spoonful of the dill sauce.
- Garnish with lemon slices and fresh dill sprigs for added flavour and presentation.

Enjoy:

- Serve the baked salmon with dill sauce immediately, accompanied by your favourite side dishes, such as roasted vegetables, steamed rice, or mixed green salad.

Nutritional Value (approx. per serving):

Calories: 300-350 calories

Protein: 30-35g

Fat: 18-20g

Carbohydrates: 3-5g

Dietary Fibre: 0g

Sugar: 1-2g

Notes

Your

Observation

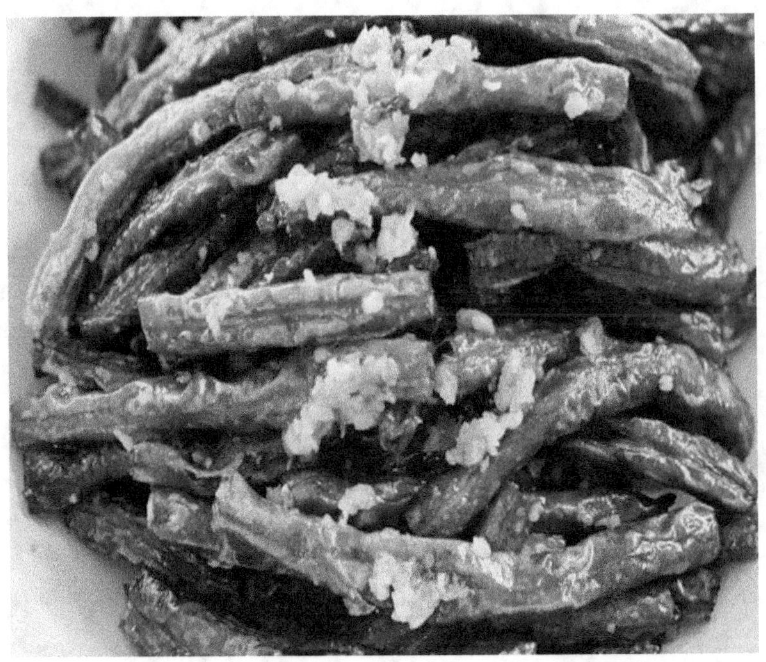

Ingredients:

- 1 pound of fresh green beans, trimmed
- 2 tablespoons of olive oil or sesame oil
- 4 cloves of minced garlic
- 1 tablespoon of soy sauce (or tamari for gluten-free option)

72

- 1 teaspoon of rice vinegar
- 1 teaspoon of honey or brown sugar (optional)
- Salt and pepper, to taste
- Red pepper flakes, for heat (optional)
- Sesame seeds, for garnish (optional)
- Sliced green onions, for garnish (optional)

Preparations:

Prepare the Green Beans:

- Rinse the green beans in cold water and blot dry with paper towels. Trim the ends and, if preferred, chop into eatable pieces.

Heat the oil:

- Heat olive or sesame oil in a large pan or wok over medium-high heat.
  Add garlic:
- Stir-fry minced garlic in a pan until fragrant, about 30 seconds. Take care

not to burn the garlic.
Stir-fry green beans:

- To stir-fry green beans, add the prepped beans to a pan. Stir-fry for 4-5 minutes, or until the green beans are soft, crisp, and brilliant green.

Season the green beans:

- In a small bowl, combine the soy sauce, rice vinegar, honey or brown sugar (if using), salt, pepper, and red pepper flakes (if using). Pour the sauce onto the green beans in the skillet. Continue Stir-fry the green beans for a further 1-2 minutes to evenly coat with the sauce.

Serve:

- Place the stir-fried garlic green beans in a serving dish. If desired, garnish with sesame seeds and thinly sliced green onions.

Enjoy:

- Serve the stir-fried garlic green beans right away as a tasty and savoury side dish to your favourite main entrée.

Nutritional Value (approx. per serving):

Calories: 80-100 calories

Protein: 2-3g

Fat: 5-7g

Carbohydrates: 8-10g

Fibre: 3-4g

Sugar: 3-4g

Notes

Your
Observation

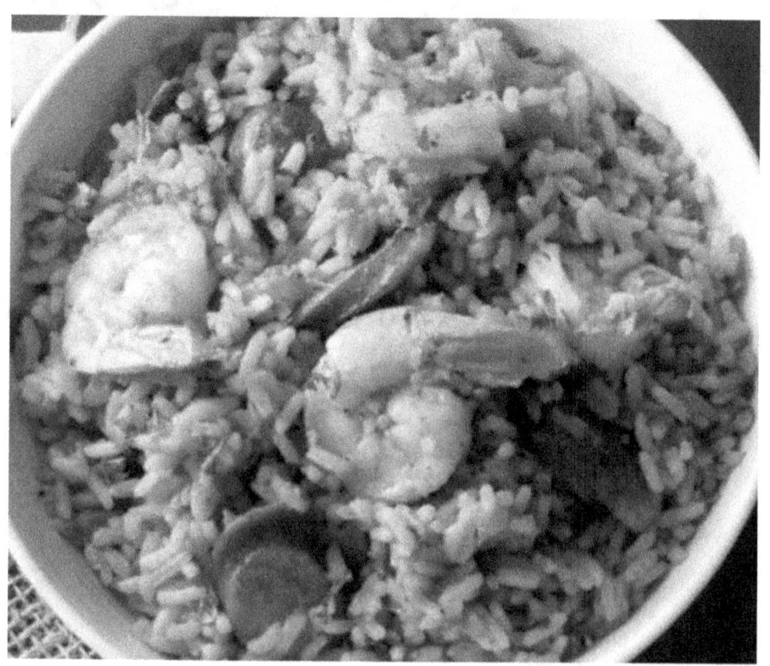

Ingredients:

- 1 pound of big shrimp, peeled and deveined
- 8 ounces of Andouille sausage, sliced

- 1 onion, chopped
- 1 bell pepper, diced
- 2 celery stalks, diced
- 3 cloves of minced garlic
- 1 can (14.5 ounces) diced tomatoes
- 1 cup of long-grain white rice
- 2 cups of chicken broth
- 1 teaspoon of Cajun seasoning
- 1/2 teaspoon of dried thyme
- 1/2 teaspoon of dried oregano
- 1/4 teaspoon of cayenne pepper (adjust to taste)
- Salt and black pepper, to taste
- 2 tablespoons olive oil
- Fresh parsley, chopped, for garnish

Preparations:

Sauté Sausage and Vegetables:

- Heat the olive oil in a large pan or Dutch oven over medium heat. Add the sliced Andouille sausage and heat for 5 minutes, or until browned.

Add the chopped onion, bell pepper, and celery to the skillet. Sauté the vegetables for 5-7 minutes, or until tender.

Add the minced garlic and simmer for another minute, or until fragrant.

Add Rice and Spices:

- Stir in rice and spices, including Cajun seasoning, dried thyme, dried oregano, cayenne pepper, salt, and black pepper. Cook the long-grain white rice for 2-3 minutes, turning regularly, until it is toasted and coated with the seasonings.

Combine Tomatoes and Broth:

- To make the sauce, combine chopped tomatoes (with liquids) and chicken stock in a pan. Stir well to combine all of the ingredients.

Simmer Jambalaya:

- Simmer To make jambalaya, bring the ingredients to a boil and then reduce to low heat. Cover and cook for 20-25 minutes, or until the rice is cooked and most of the liquid has been absorbed. Stir occasionally to avoid sticking.

Add shrimp:

- When rice is almost cooked, add peeled and deveined prawns to the pan. Cook for 4-5 minutes, or until prawns are pink and opaque.

Garnish and serve:

- Remove the skillet from the heat. Top the shrimp and sausage jambalaya with chopped fresh   parsley.
  Serve hot and relish this tasty and soothing meal.

Nutritional Value (approx. per serving):

Calories: 350-400 kcal

Protein: 25-30g

Fat: 15-20g

Carbohydrates: 30-35g

Fibre: 3-5g

Sugar: 3-5g

Notes

Your

Observation

CHAPTER 6: SNACKS AND SIDES

Truffle Rosemary Nuts

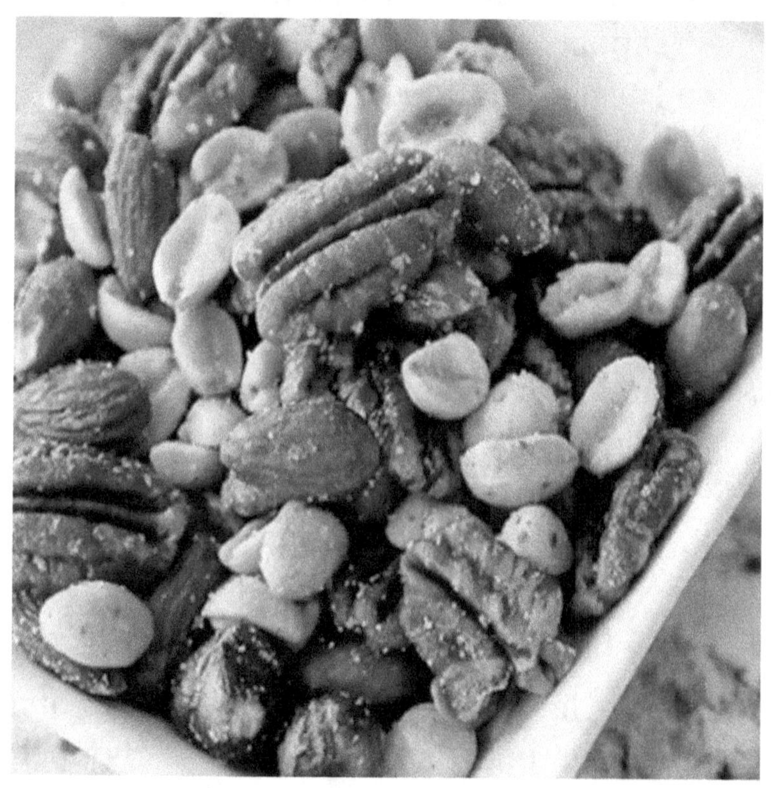

Ingredients:

- 2 cups of mixed nuts (such as almonds, cashews, pecans, walnuts)
- 1 tablespoon of truffle oil
- 1 tablespoon of olive oil
- 2 teaspoons of fresh rosemary, thinly chopped
- 1 teaspoon of garlic powder
- 1 teaspoon of onion powder
- 1/2 teaspoon of salt (adjust to taste)
- 1/4 teaspoon of black pepper

Preparations:

Preheat the Oven:

- Preheat the oven to 325°F (160° C). Line a baking sheet with parchment or aluminium foil.

Prepare the nuts:

- In a large mixing bowl, add the nuts, truffle oil, olive oil, finely chopped rosemary, garlic powder, onion powder, salt, and black pepper. Toss the nuts until they are uniformly covered with the   seasoning.

Spread on Baking Sheet:

- Spread seasoned nuts in a single layer on a preheated baking sheet.

Bake the   nuts:

- Bake the nuts in a preheated oven for 15-20 minutes, stirring regularly, until golden brown and aromatic. Keep an eye on them to avoid burning

Cool:

- Remove the baking sheet from the oven and allow nuts to cool fully. As they cool, they will get cripsy.

Serve:

- To serve or store, place the cooled truffle rosemary nuts in an airtight container or serving bowl. Serve as a tasty snack or appetiser.

Nutritional Value (approx. per serving):

Calories: 180-200 kcal

Protein: 5-7g

Fat: 15-18g

Carbohydrates: 7-9g

Fiber: 2-3g

Sugar: 1-2g

Sodium: 50-100g

Notes

Your

Observation

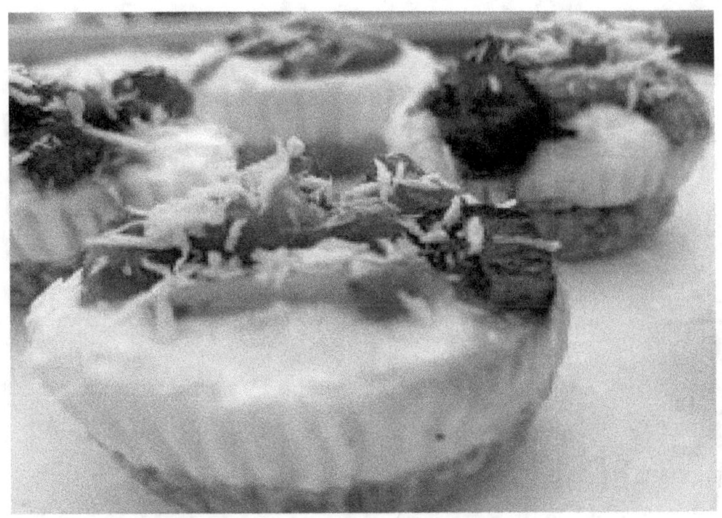

Ingredients:

- 2 cups of granola (purchased or homemade)
- 1/4 cup of honey or maple syrup
- 2 tablespoons of coconut oil, melted
- 1 cup of Greek yogurt (plain or flavoured)

- 1/2 cup of fresh berries (such as strawberries, blueberries, or raspberries)
- Optional: shredded coconut, chopped nuts, or chocolate chips for topping

Preparations:

Prepare Granola Mixture:

- In a mixing dish, combine the granola, honey, maple syrup, and melted coconut oil. Stir until thoroughly blended and the granola is uniformly covered.

Form Granola   Cups:

- Line the muffin tray with silicone or paper liners. Spoon the granola mixture into each muffin cup, pushing it firmly into the bottom and up the sides to create a cup shape. Make careful to leave a little depression in the middle of each cup.

Fill with yoghurt and berries:

- Spoon Greek yoghurt into each granola cup, almost to the top. Top with fresh berries and any other toppings you choose, such as shredded coconut, chopped almonds, or chocolate chips.

Freeze:

- Freeze the muffin pan for 2-3 hours to firm up the granola cups.

Serve:

- To serve, just remove the frozen granola cups from the muffin pan. Allow them to remain at room temperature for a few minutes to soften before serving.

Enjoy:

- These frozen granola cups make a delicious and healthful snack or dessert.

Keep any leftovers in an airtight jar in the freezer for later use.

Nutritional Value (approx. per serving):

Calories: 150-200 kcal

Protein: 3-5g

Fat: 8-10g

Carbohydrates: 15-20g

Fibre: 2-3g

Sugar: 8-12g

Sodium: 20-50mg

Notes

Your

Observation

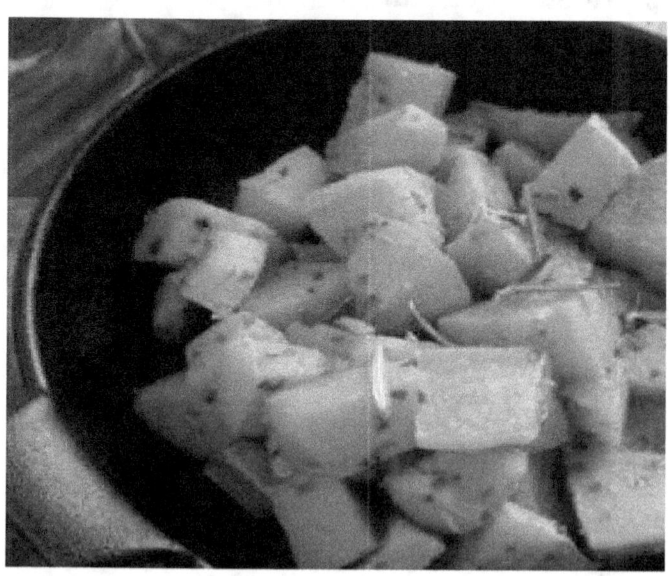

Ingredients:

- 2 average-size sweet potatoes, peeled and diced
- 1 onion, thinly chopped
- 2 cloves of minced garlic
- 1 tablespoon fresh ginger, grated
- 1 can of (14 ounces) coconut milk
- 1 can of (14.5 ounces) diced tomatoes

- 1 can of (15 ounces) chickpeas, rinsed and drained
- 2 cups of vegetable broth
- 1 tablespoon of curry powder
- 1 teaspoon of ground cumin
- 1 teaspoon of ground turmeric
- 1/2 teaspoon of ground coriander
- 1/4 teaspoon of cayenne pepper (optional, for heat)
- Salt and pepper, to taste
- 2 tablespoons of olive oil or coconut oil
- Fresh cilantro, chopped, for garnish
- Cooked rice or naan bread, for serving

Preparations:

Sauté Onion, Garlic, and Ginger:

- In a large saucepan or Dutch oven, warm the olive or coconut oil over medium heat. Sauté the chopped onion until softened, about 3-4 minutes. Add the minced garlic and grated ginger and simmer for another 1-2 minutes, or until fragrant.

Add spices:

- Add the curry powder, cumin, turmeric, coriander, and cayenne pepper (if using) to the saucepan. Stir thoroughly to coat the onion combination with spices, then fry for 1-2 minutes to toast them.

Cook sweet potatoes:

- Stir in the diced sweet potatoes and spice mixture until well combined.

Simmer with liquid ingredients:

- Pour in the coconut milk, chopped tomatoes (with their juices), and veggie broth. Stir in the drained and rinsed chickpeas. Season with salt and pepper to taste.

Simmer the curry:

- Bring the mixture to a boil, then turn the heat down to low. Cover the saucepan and heat for 20-25 minutes, or until the sweet potatoes are soft and fully cooked. Stir occasionally to avoid sticking.

Adjust seasoning:

- Taste the curry and adjust the spice as required. Add extra salt, pepper, or spices to taste.

Serve:

- Serve the sweet potato curry hot and garnish with chopped fresh cilantro. For a complete and fulfilling dinner, serve over cooked rice or over naan bread.

Nutritional Value (approx. per serving):

Calories: 250-300 kcal

Protein: 6-8g

Fat: 10-12g

Carbohydrates: 35-40g

Fibre: 6-8g

Sugar: 8-10g

Sodium: 500-600 mg

Notes

Your Observation

CHAPTER 7: DESSERTS OPTIONS

Raspberry Chia Pudding

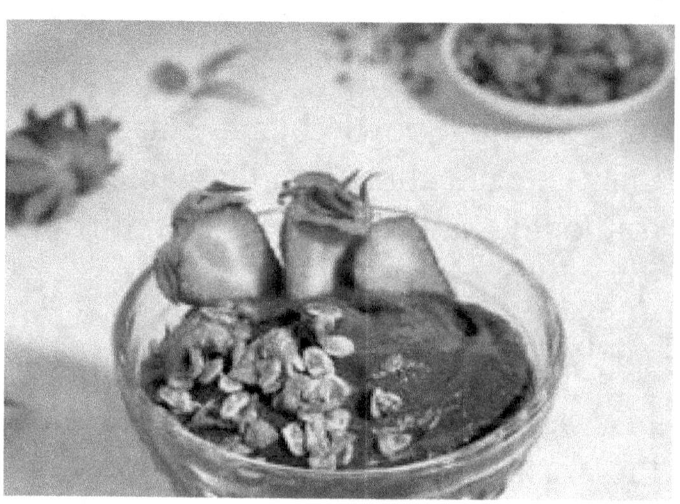

Ingredients:

- 1/4 cup of chia seeds
- 1 cup of unsweetened almond milk (or any preferred one)
- 1 tablespoon of maple syrup or honey (adjust to taste)

- 1/2 teaspoon of vanilla extract
- 1/2 cup of fresh raspberries (or frozen, thawed)
- Additional raspberries and mint leaves for garnish (optional)

Preparations:

Prepare Chia Seed Mixture:

- In a mixing bowl, blend chia seeds, unsweetened almond milk, maple syrup (or honey), and vanilla extract. Stir well to mix.

Mash raspberries:

- In a separate dish, using a fork, mash the fresh raspberries until smooth. If using frozen raspberries, be careful to defrost them before mashing.

Layer the pudding:

- Divide the chia seed mixture evenly into serving glasses or jars, filling them approximately halfway.

Add Raspberry Layer:

- Divide the chia seed mixture evenly between the glasses and top with a layer of crushed raspberries.

Top with the remaining chia seed mixture:

- Pour the remaining chia seed mixture over the raspberry layer in each glass, filling them to the top.

Chill:

- Cover the glasses or jars with plastic wrap or lids and chill for at least 2-3 hours, ideally overnight, to allow the chia seeds to absorb liquid and thicken.

Garnish and serve:

- When the raspberry chia pudding has chilled and set, decorate with fresh raspberries and mint leaves, if preferred. Serve chilled and enjoy

Nutritional Value (approx. per serving):

Calories: 150-200 kcal

Protein: 4-6g

Fat: 8-10g

Carbohydrates: 15-20g

Fibre: 8-10g

Sugar: 6-8g

Sodium: 50-100mg

Notes

Your

Observation

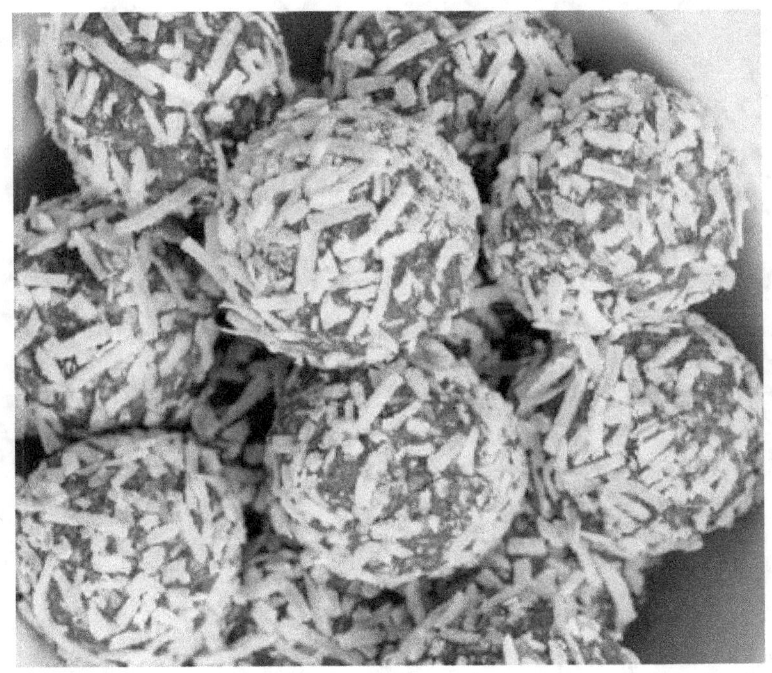

Ingredients:

- 1/2 cup dried raspberries (alternatively cranberries)
- 1/2 cup of frozen raspberries
- 1/3 cup of almond meal

- 1/2 cup of cashews
- 1/4 cup of cashew butter
- 1 cup of shredded coconut, (add extra to roll in)
- 1/2 tbsp of Tropeaka Immunity Powder
- 1 tbsp of Tropeaka Camu Camu Powder
- 6 Medjool dates, pitted

Preparations:

Prepare Cashews:

- If your cashews are not soft yet, soak them in water for a few hours or overnight. Drain and rinse them before using.

Blend cashews:

- In a food processor, combine the soaked cashews and pulse until finely crushed to a meal-like consistency.

Combine Ingredients:

- Put the frozen raspberries, dried raspberries (or cranberries), almond flour, cashew butter, shredded coconut, Tropeaka Immunity Powder, Tropeaka Camu Camu Powder, and pitted Medjool dates in the food processor.

Blend the mixture:

- In a food processor, pulse the ingredients until fully incorporated and the mixture resembles a sticky dough. Stop and scrape the sides of the food processor as needed to ensure that all ingredients are equally distributed.

Form Bliss Balls:

- Once the mixture has reached the proper consistency, scoop out pieces using a tablespoon. Roll each part between your palms to make balls.

Roll in coconut:

- Roll the created bliss balls in shredded coconut until thoroughly covered. This stage adds texture and improves the flavour.

Chill:

- Transfer the coated bliss balls to a dish or baking sheet lined with parchment paper. Place them in the refrigerator to cool for at least 30 minutes. Chilling helps the bliss balls stiffen up and maintain their form.

Serve and enjoy:

- Once cooled, the Berry Bliss Balls are ready to eat. Refrigerate any leftovers in an airtight container for up to a week.

Nutritional Value (approx. per serving):

Calories: 120-140 kcal

Protein: 2-3g

Fat: 7-9g

Carbohydrates: 12-15g

Fibre: 2-3g

Sugar: 8-10g

Sodium: 5-10mg

Notes

Your

Observation

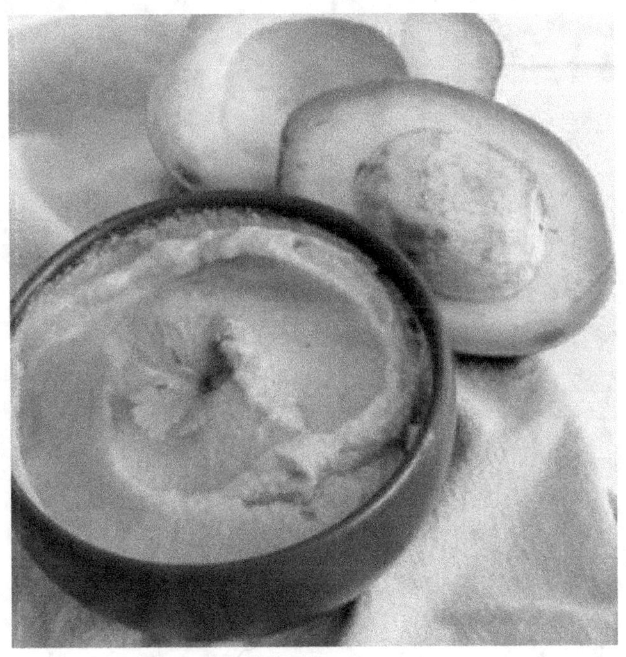

Ingredients:

- 2 ripe avocados
- 1/4 cup of unsweetened cocoa powder
- 1/4 cup of maple syrup or honey (adjust to taste)
- 1 teaspoon of vanilla extract

- Pinch of salt
- Optional toppings: whipped cream, fresh berries, shaved chocolate

Preparations:

Prepare Avocados:

- Cut the avocados in halves, remove the pits, and transfer the flesh to a blender or food processor.

Add cocoa powder and sweetener:

- In a blender, combine the unsweetened cocoa powder, maple syrup or honey, vanilla essence, and a sprinkle of salt with the avocado flesh.

Blend until smooth:

- Blend the ingredients until smooth and creamy, scraping down the sides of the blender or food processor as required to ensure thorough mixing.

Taste and adjust:

- Taste the avocado chocolate mousse and adjust the sweetness and cocoa strength to your liking. If desired, add extra maple syrup or chocolate powder.

Chill (optional):

- Transfer the avocado chocolate mousse to a bowl or individual serving plates and refrigerate in the refrigerator for at least 30 minutes before serving.

Serve and garnish:

- After chilling (if preferred), serve the avocado chocolate mousse in dishes or glasses. To add a finishing touch, top each serving with whipped cream, fresh berries, or shaved chocolate.

Enjoy:

This creamy and rich avocado chocolate mousse makes an excellent treat or snack!

Nutritional Value (approx. per serving):

Calories: 150-200 kcal

Protein: 2-3g

Fat: 10-15g

Carbohydrates: 15-20g

Fibre: 5-7g

Sugar: 8-12g

Sodium: 5-10 mg

Notes

Your
Observation

CHAPTER 8: BEVERAGES

Herbal Teas and Infusions

Peppermint Tea: Known for its refreshing and minty flavour, peppermint tea is often enjoyed for its soothing properties, helping to alleviate digestive discomfort and promote relaxation.

Chamomile Tea: Chamomile tea is prized for its gentle, floral taste and calming effects. It is commonly consumed before bedtime to promote relaxation and improve sleep quality.

Ginger Tea: With its warming and spicy flavour, ginger tea is favoured for its potential digestive benefits, helping to alleviate nausea, indigestion, and bloating.

Lemon Balm Tea: Lemon balm tea has a mild citrus flavour and is often used to reduce stress, promote relaxation, and improve mood.

Hibiscus Tea: Hibiscus tea has a tart and tangy flavour, reminiscent of cranberries. It is rich in antioxidants and may help lower blood pressure and improve heart health.

Lavender Infusion: Lavender infusion offers a delicate floral aroma and is commonly used to promote relaxation, reduce anxiety, and improve sleep quality.

Nettle Tea: Nettle tea has a grassy and earthy flavour and is believed to offer various health benefits, including relieving allergy symptoms, supporting kidney function, and reducing inflammation.

Preparation:

To prepare herbal teas and infusions, simply steep the desired herbs, spices, flowers, or fruits in hot water for several minutes. Strain the mixture before serving and sweeten with honey or other sweeteners if desired. Herbal teas can also be enjoyed cold by brewing them in hot water first and then allowing them to cool before refrigerating or serving over ice.

Green Goddess Smoothie

Ingredients:

- 1 cup of spinach
- 1/2 cup of kale
- 1/2 cucumber, peeled and cut
- 1/2 avocado
- 1 banana
- 1 tablespoon of chia seeds
- 1 cup of unsweetened almond milk

Preparations:

- In a blender, blend all ingredients until smooth and creamy. Add additional almond milk as needed to get the desired consistency. Serve cold.

Nutritional Value (approx. per serving):

Calories: 200-250 kcal

Protein: 5-7g

Fat: 12-15g

Carbohydrates: 20-25g

Fibre: 6-8g

Sugar: 10-12g

Tropical Paradise Smoothie

Ingredients:

- 1/2 cup of pineapple chunks
- 1/2 banana
- 1/4 cup of mango chunks
- 1/4 cup of Greek yogurt
- 1 tablespoon of coconut flakes
- 1 tablespoon of hemp seeds
- 1/2 cup of coconut water

Preparations:

- In a blender, blend all of the ingredients until smooth and creamy. If necessary, add additional coconut water to get the desired consistency. If desired, garnish with extra coconut flakes.

Nutritional Value (approx. per serving):

Calories: 200-250 kcal

Protein: 4-6g

Fat: 8-10g

Carbohydrates: 30-35g

Fibre: 4-6g

Sugar: 20-25g

Creamy Peanut Butter Banana Smoothie

Ingredients:

- 1 ripe banana
- 2 tablespoons of peanut butter
- 1/4 cup of rolled oats
- 1 tablespoon of flaxseed meal
- 1 tablespoon of honey or maple syrup
- 1 cup of unsweetened almond milk

Preparations:

- Combine all ingredients in a blender and blend until smooth. Add additional almond milk as needed to get the desired consistency. This protein-rich smoothie makes a great breakfast or post-workout snack.

Nutritional Value (approx. per serving):

Calories: 300-350 kcal

Protein: 8-10g

Fat: 12-15g

Carbohydrates: 40-45g

Fibre: 6-8g

Sugar: 15-20g

Notes

Your

Observation

Hydration Tips for CRPS Patients

Hydration is essential for everyone, but it is especially critical for those with CRPS (Complex Regional Pain Syndrome) since it can affect circulation, nerve function, and general well-being. Here are some hydration strategies geared especially for CRPS patients:

Drink Plenty of Water: Aim to consume at least eight 8-ounce glasses of water each day, or more if you are physically active or live in a hot region. Proper hydration improves blood flow, regulates body temperature, and promotes general health.

Consider Electrolyte Balance: CRPS sufferers may benefit from keeping correct electrolyte balance, as imbalances can worsen symptoms like muscular cramping and exhaustion. Include electrolyte-rich foods and beverages in your diet, such as coconut water, bananas, leafy greens, and sports drinks (preferably low in sugar and salt).

Avoid Excess Caffeine and Alcohol: Caffeine and alcohol can both cause dehydration and increase symptoms in CRPS sufferers. Limit your consumption of caffeinated beverages such as coffee, tea, and soda, as well as alcoholic beverages, and be sure to drink enough of water.

Monitor Medication Side Effects: Some CRPS treatments may raise the risk of dehydration. Be aware of these potential side effects and take actions to mitigate them, such as drinking more water or visiting your healthcare professional if necessary.

Consume Water-Rich items: Add hydrating items to your diet, such as fruits and vegetables high in water content. Examples include watermelon, cucumber, oranges, strawberries, and lettuce. These meals not only help with hydration, but they also include critical vitamins, minerals, and antioxidants.

Set Hydration Reminders: It is easy to forget to drink enough water during the day, especially if you are experiencing chronic pain or discomfort. To help you keep hydrated on a continuous basis, use phone reminders or establish specified times to drink water.

Listen to Your Body: Pay attention to your body's indications of thirst and hydration. Thirst is a clear indication that your body requires more water, so pay attention to it and drink plenty of water throughout the day.

Be Aware of Fluid Loss: CRPS symptoms such as sweating, restricted movement, and diminished feeling can all increase fluid loss and dehydration risk. Take particular measures to restore fluids lost via perspiration and evaporation when exercising, in hot weather, or in times of heightened discomfort.

CHAPTER 9: 10 DAY MEAL PLAN

Breakfast: Açaí Smoothie Bowl

Lunch: Grilled chicken salad with mixed greens, cherry tomatoes, cucumbers, and balsamic vinaigrette

Dinner: Baked salmon with roasted sweet potatoes and steamed broccoli

Day 2

Breakfast: Frittata muffins

Lunch: Quinoa salad with chickpeas, roasted vegetables, and lemon-tahini dressing

Dinner: Turkey chili with kidney beans, corn, and diced tomatoes, served with whole grain cornbread

Day 3:

Breakfast: Banana oatmeal topped with almond butter and sliced strawberries

Lunch: Gluten-free Mujaddara

Dinner: Stir-fried tofu with mixed vegetables and brown rice

Day 4:

Breakfast: Smoothie bowl with spinach, mixed berries, banana, and almond milk, topped with granola and sliced almonds

Lunch: Lentil soup with carrots, celery, and spinach, served with whole grain bread

Dinner: Grilled shrimp skewers with quinoa pilaf and roasted asparagus

Day 5:

Breakfast: Whole grain pancakes with Greek yogurt and sliced peaches

Lunch: Turkey and avocado wrap with lettuce, tomato, and whole grain tortilla

Dinner: Baked chicken breast with mashed cauliflower and sautéed green beans

Day 6:

Breakfast: Vegetables scramble with eggs, bell peppers, onions, and mushrooms

Lunch: Mediterranean quinoa salad with cucumber, cherry tomatoes, olives, and feta cheese

Dinner: Spaghetti squash with marinara sauce and turkey meatballs, served with a side salad

Day 7:

Breakfast: Overnight oats with almond milk, chia seeds, and mixed berries

Lunch: Crispy potatoes with kefir and vegetables

Dinner: Beef stir-fry with broccoli, bell peppers, and snap peas, served over brown rice

Day 8:

Breakfast: Whole grain toast with mashed avocado and poached eggs

Lunch: Kale and cranberry salad with grilled chicken, almonds, and citrus vinaigrette

Dinner: Baked cod with lemon-dill sauce, roasted potatoes, and steamed green beans

Breakfast: Smoothie with spinach, pineapple, banana, Greek yogurt, and almond milk

Lunch: Quinoa and black bean salad with roasted corn, bell peppers, and cilantro-lime dressing

Dinner: Vegetable curry with chickpeas, cauliflower, and spinach, served with brown rice

Breakfast: Greek yogurt with honey, sliced almonds, and mixed berries

Lunch: Grilled vegetable panini with hummus on whole grain bread

Dinner: Stuffed bell peppers with ground turkey, quinoa, and diced tomatoes, served with a side of roasted Brussels sprouts

CHAPTER 10:
CONCLUSION

In a nutshell, the creation and execution of a CRPS (difficult Regional Pain Syndrome) cookbook provides a holistic approach to managing this difficult ailment. By focusing on nutrition customised to the specific needs of CRPS sufferers, such a cookbook is an invaluable resource for anyone dealing with chronic pain and inflammation. The CRPS cookbook encourages both physical and emotional well-being via carefully picked dishes and nutritional instructions.

This cookbook enables CRPS patients to take charge of their health and learn about the possible advantages of a well-balanced, nutrient-dense diet. Individuals with CRPS can improve their nutritional intake by integrating anti-inflammatory components, hydrating foods, and meals designed to promote general wellness. Furthermore, the cookbook promotes a sense of community and support among CRPS patients by offering a forum for sharing experiences, recipes, and ideas into managing the illness.

In summary, the CRPS cookbook takes a comprehensive approach to wellbeing, recognising the interdependence of diet, pain management, and quality of life. As part of a holistic treatment plan, the cookbook is an invaluable resource for CRPS sufferers and carers, providing practical advice and inspiration for nourishing the body, mind, and spirit in the face of hardship.

STAY HEALTHY!

Bonus

MEAL
PLANNER
DAILY
DATE
BREAKFAST
NOTES
LUNCH
SNACK
ITEMS LIST
DINNER

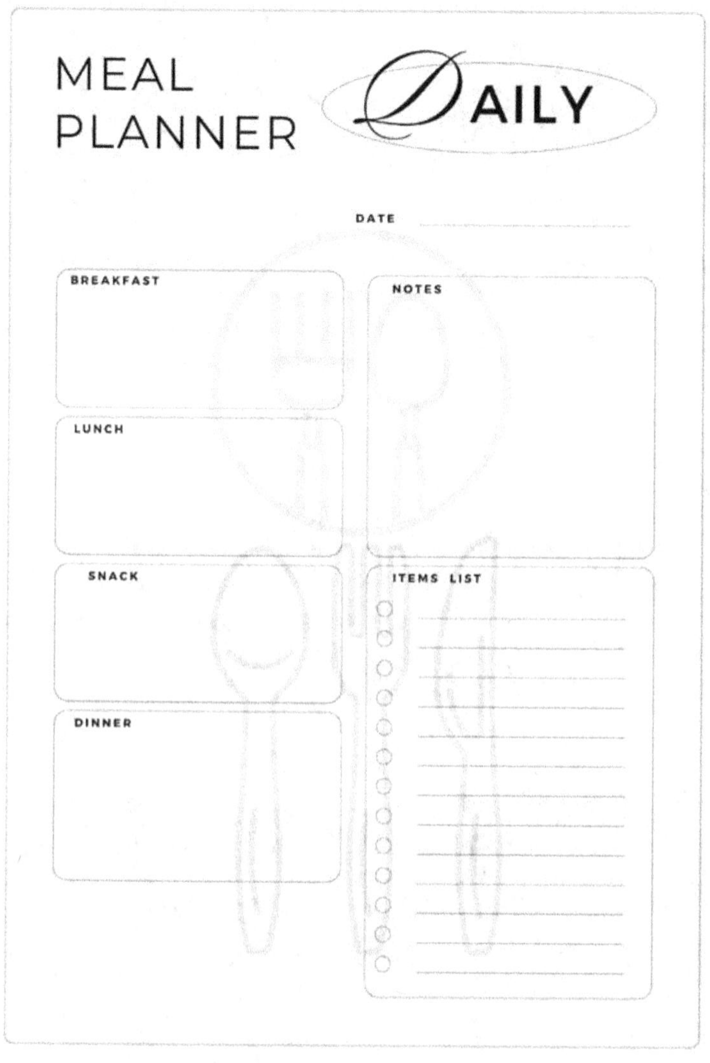

MEAL PLANNER

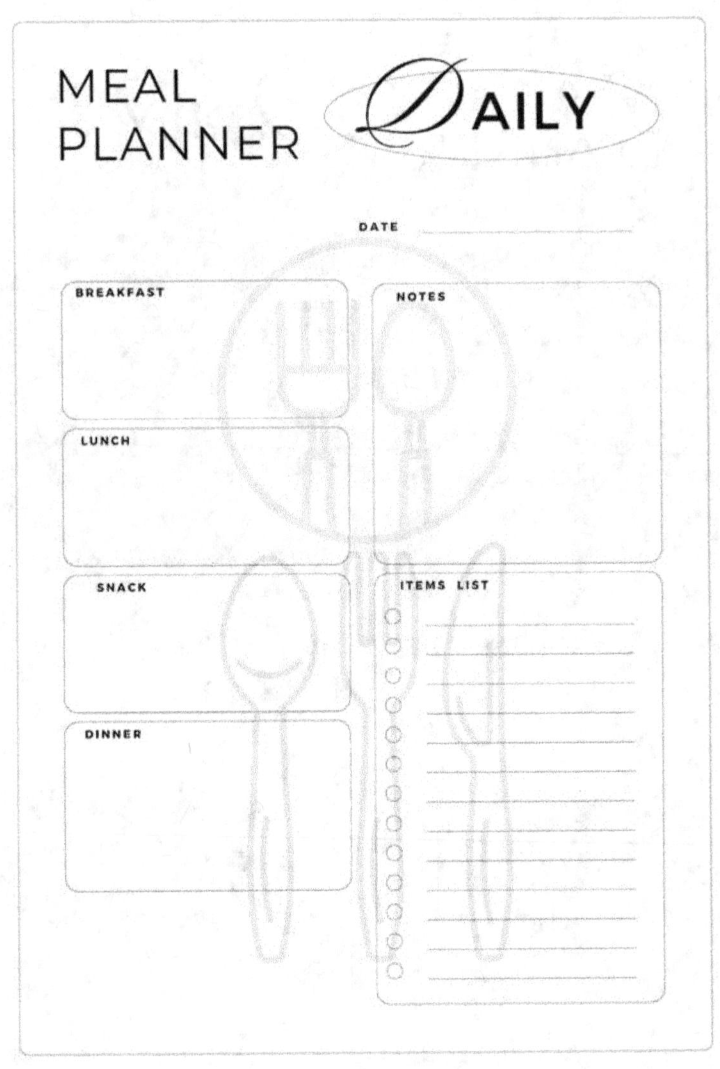

MEAL PLANNER

DAILY

DATE

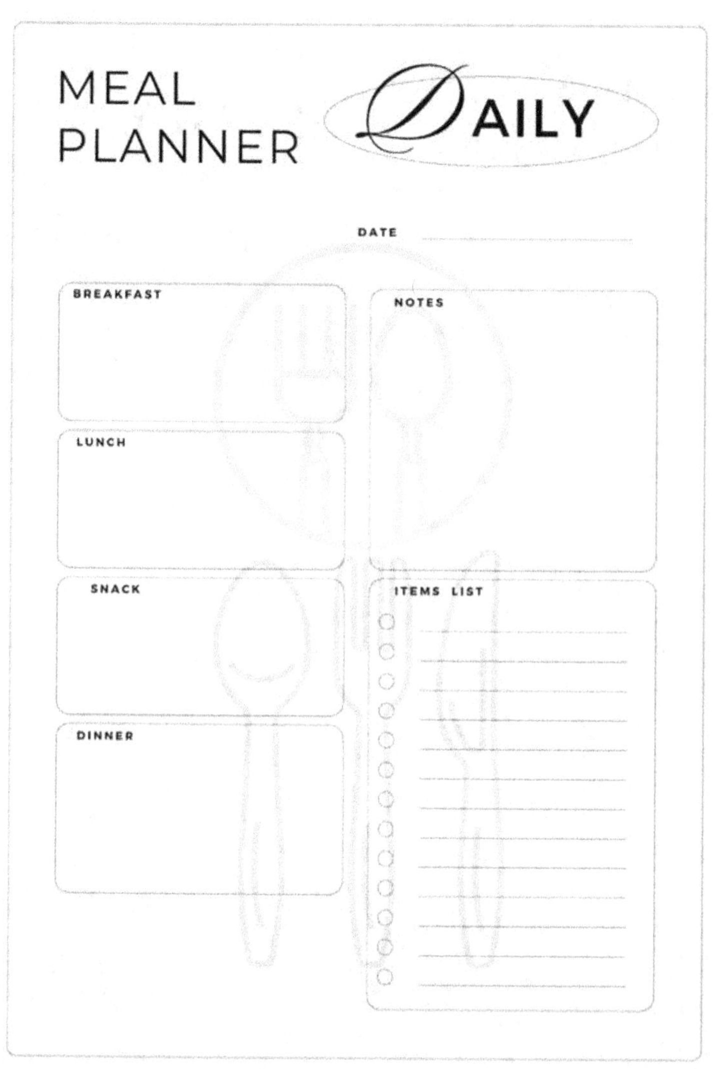

BREAKFAST

LUNCH

SNACK

DINNER

NOTES

ITEMS LIST

MEAL PLANNER

DAILY

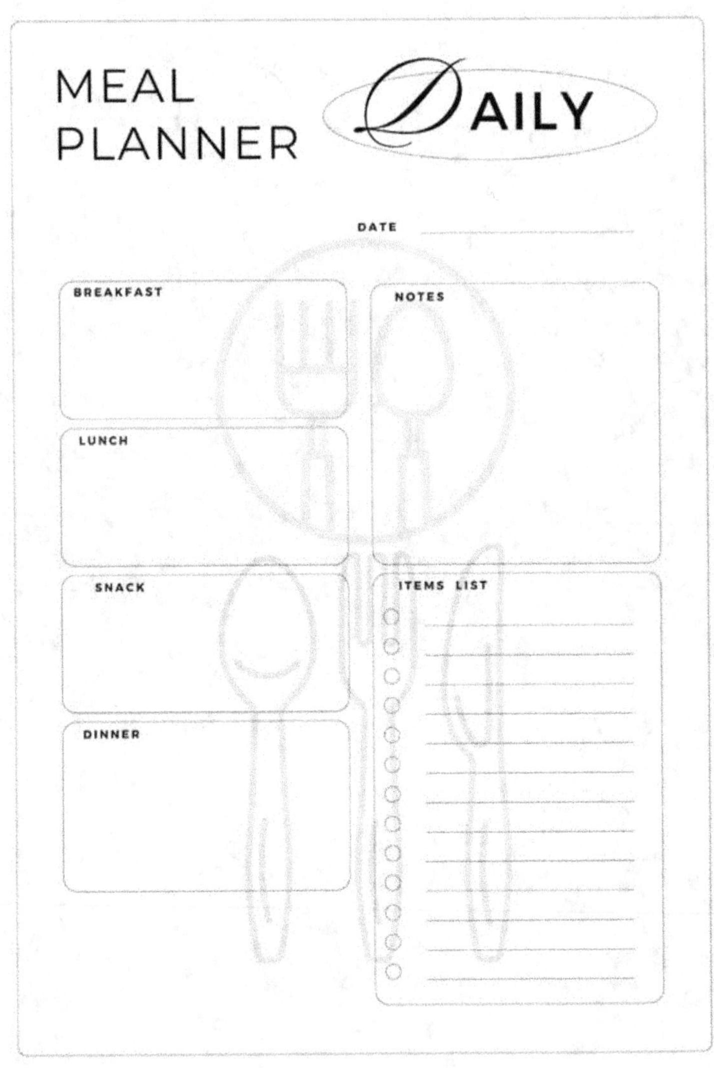

DATE

BREAKFAST

LUNCH

SNACK

DINNER

NOTES

ITEMS LIST

MEAL PLANNER

DAILY

DATE

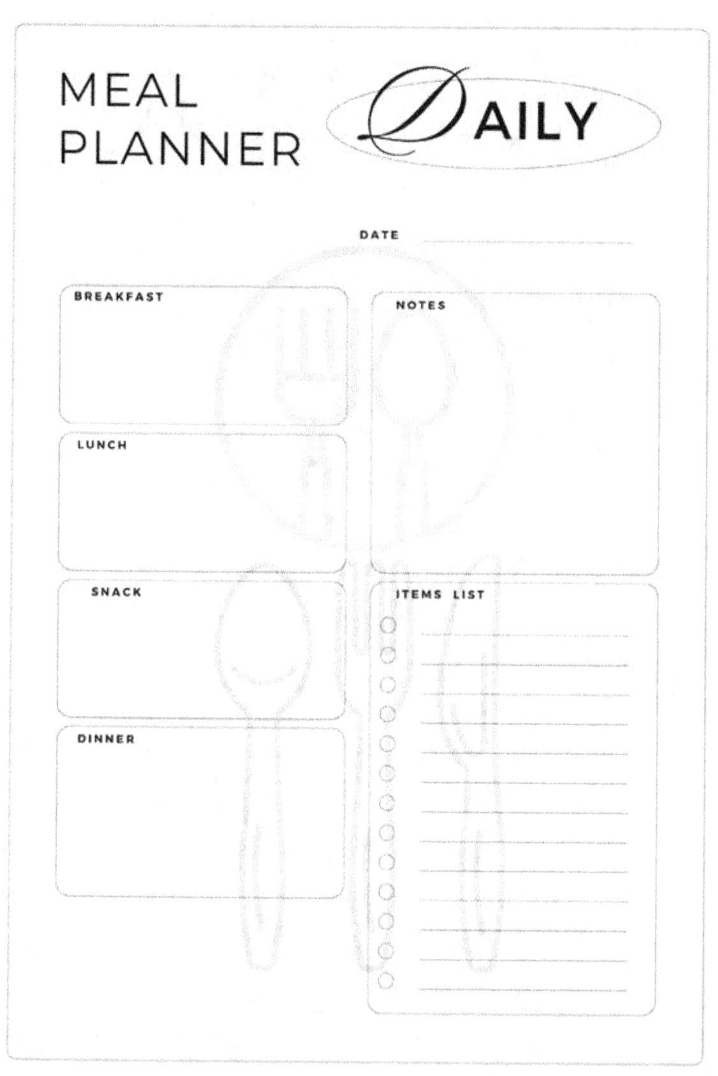

BREAKFAST

NOTES

LUNCH

SNACK

ITEMS LIST

DINNER

MEAL PLANNER

DAILY

DATE

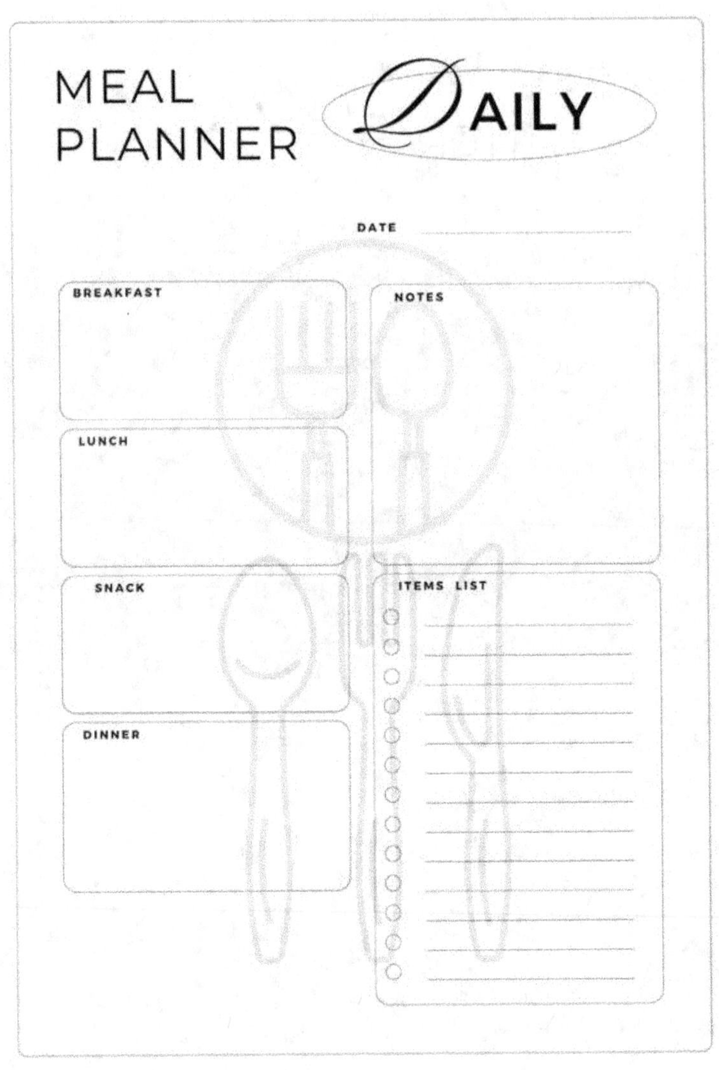

BREAKFAST

LUNCH

SNACK

DINNER

NOTES

ITEMS LIST

MEAL PLANNER

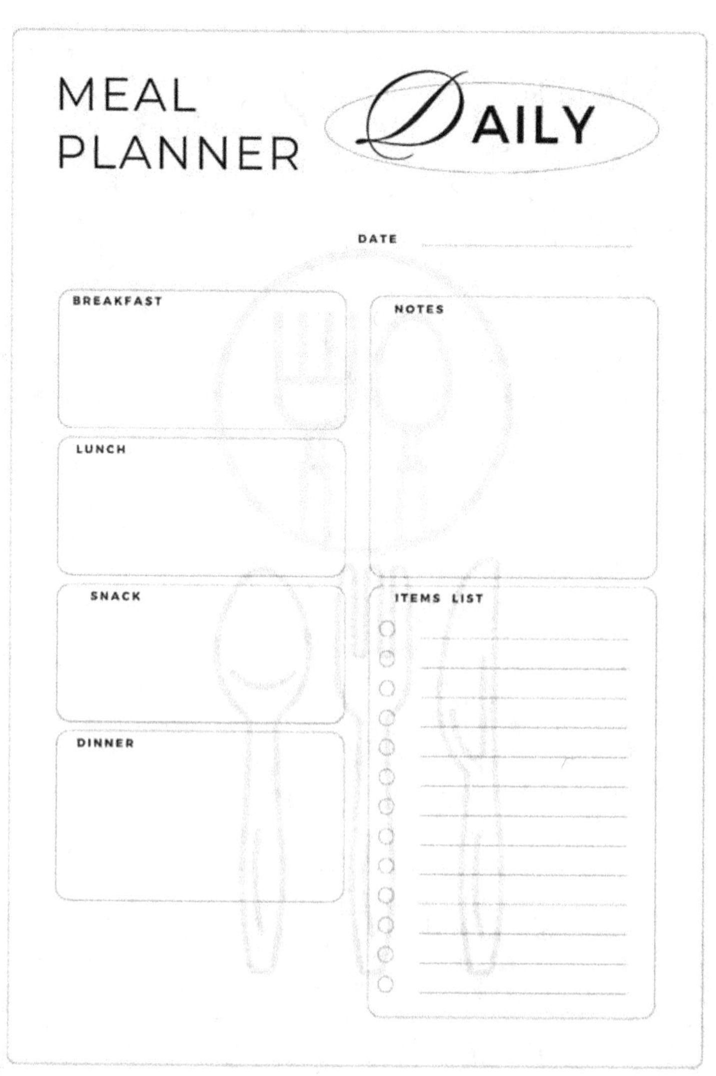

DAILY

DATE

BREAKFAST

NOTES

LUNCH

SNACK

ITEMS LIST

DINNER

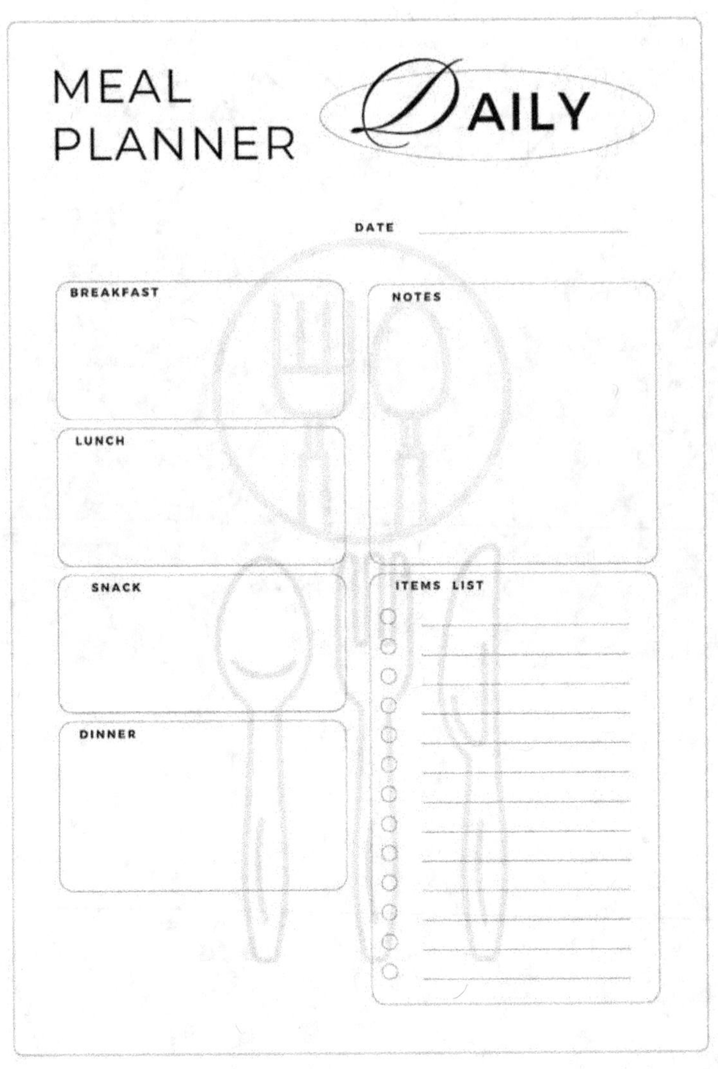

MEAL
PLANNER

DAILY

DATE

BREAKFAST

LUNCH

SNACK

DINNER

NOTES

ITEMS LIST

MEAL PLANNER

DAILY

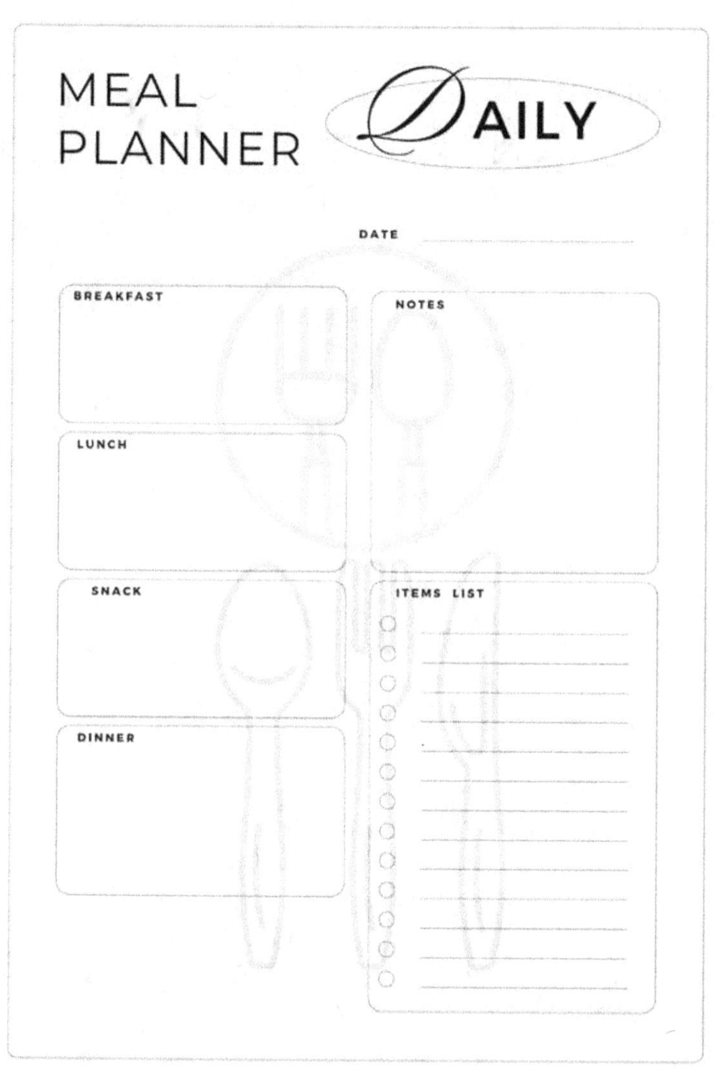

DATE

BREAKFAST

LUNCH

SNACK

DINNER

NOTES

ITEMS LIST

MEAL PLANNER

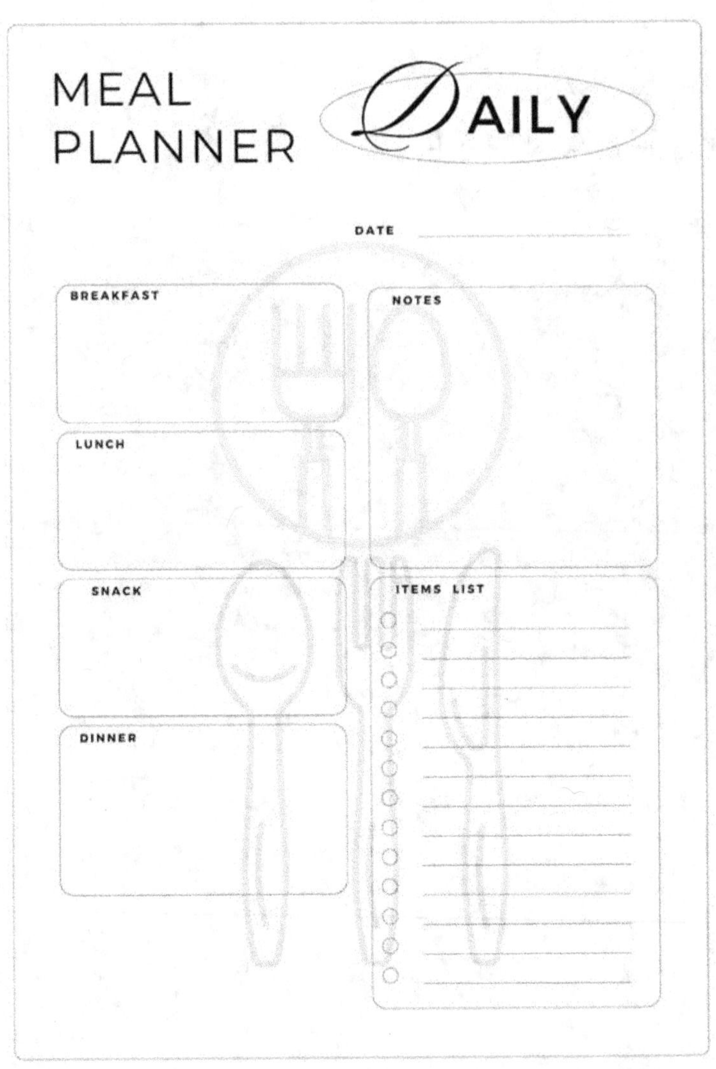